THE ATKINS DIET

COOKBOOK

FOR

NEWBIES AND BEGINNERS

BY

Dr. Christen Zimmermann

© COPYRIGHT

Table of Contents

INTRODUCTION

Does bacon and eggs for breakfast, smoked salmon with cream cheese for lunch, and steak cooked in butter for dinner sound like a weight-loss menu too good to be true? If you love foods like these and aren't a fan of carrot-filled diets, Atkins may be right for you.

WHAT IS THE ATKINS DIET?

The Atkins diet is similar to a ketogenic diet as both emphasise the consumption of fat and protein but severely restrict carbohydrates. The body will turn to glycogen stores (carbohydrates) for energy first if supplies are plentiful. Ketogenic diets essentially force the body to switch from burning carbohydrates for energy to burning fat. This often has the desirable effect of weight loss, though high levels of ketones in the body can be problematic and may lead to a state known as ketoacidosis.

THE HISTORY OF ATKINS

The daddy of low-carb diets, Robert Atkins may not have been the first to harness the appeal of carb-free, but he was certainly the first to bring the concept to the mainstream dieting public.

In 1963, American physician and cardiologist Robert Atkins came across a study published by Dr Alfred W. Pennington. His research explored the theory that cutting starch and sugar from the diet could lead to significant weight loss. Putting the pound-shedding theory to the test, Atkins shrunk his own bulk and adapted the findings into the diet and formidable brand we know today.

Since his first book, 'Dr Atkins diet revolution', was published in 1972 the waist-reducing formulae has been nipped and tucked into an increasingly modern form. To date, Atkins diet books have sold in the region of 15 million copies – making it the bestselling weight loss book in history.

The four phases of Atkins summarised from atkins.com:

1) The induction phase of the programme starts by cutting carbs almost completely from your daily diet. In fact, you are encouraged to only eat 20g of net carbs a day – compared to the government guidelines (Reference Intake) of 260g.

The aim here is to get your body to rely primarily on fats for energy. Followers will lose the majority of weight in this phase and eat this way for at least two weeks.

2) The second stage focuses on continued weight loss and you are now allowed between 25 and 45 grams of net carbs a day. The idea is to slowly re-introduce carbohydrates back into your diet to avoid weight gain.

3) The pre-maintenance stage continues to re-introduce carbs back into the diet, with five main objectives for dieters including losing the last '10 pounds' slowly, testing your tolerance for previously forbidden foods and maintaining previous weight loss. Once you've maintained your goal weight for a month you're ready to move onto stage four…

4) This final, lifelong phase is billed simply as maintenance. Atkins suggests that by now you should have discovered how many carbohydrates you can include in your diet without regaining weight.

Smoked Salmon Poke Bites

Ingredients:

• Seasoned rice crackers

• 1 cup cooked sushi or jasmine rice

• Pickled cucumbers (see below)

• 4 ounces smoked salmon, cut into small sizes

• Sliced avocado

• Pickled ginger

• Finely diced red onion

• Sesame oil, for drizzling

• Soy sauce or coconut aminos, for drizzling

Pickled Cucumbers:

• 1 large cucumber

• 2 teaspoons rice vinegar

• 1 teaspoon sugar

Directions:

1. Using a vegetable peeler, thinly peel cucumber into strips, excluding the seed center.

2. To pickle the cucumbers, add sliced cucumber into a small bowl along with rice vinegar and sugar, and toss to coat. Let marinate for at least ten minutes.

3. To layer the bites, gently add a spoonful of cooked rice to the top of the cracker. Next, add pickled cucumbers folded on top, then a piece of smoked salmon, sliced avocado, and pickled ginger, and top with diced red onion. Continue until all crackers are layered.

4. For extra flavor, drizzle a small amount of sesame oil and soy sauce on top of each layered bite.

5. Pro tip: Toss any extra ingredients into a bowl to make a poke bowl you can enjoy for lunch!

These bacon-wrapped sweet potatoes are so versatile, you can serve them before your meal, on the side, or even for breakfast on the morning of Thanksgiving. Delicious and Paleo-approved, they really have no downsides.

Ingredients:

• 3 medium sweet potatoes

• 20 slices bacon

• 1/4 teaspoon pink salt

• Freshly ground pepper

Directions:

1. Preheat oven to 400 degrees F.

2. Line a baking sheet with parchment paper.

3. Cut sweet potatoes into thick cut wedges or fry shapes.

4. Wrap each sweet potato with a piece of bacon, slightly overlapping the bacon on itself as it goes around the sweet potato.

5. Place the sweet potatoes in a single layer onto the baking sheet, leaving an inch or two in between each one. Do in two batches if needed. Sprinkle salt and pepper on top.

6. Bake for 35 minutes. Sweet potatoes should be tender and bacon crispy.

7. Serve with ketchup, ranch, or aioli.

Next up on our need-to-make-immediately list is Koufteh Ghelgheli, an Iranian dish comprised of lamb meatballs with carrots, potatoes, and overall deliciousness. A hearty and warm-you-to-your-toes kind of meal, this Middle Eastern recipe should definitely be in your weekly rotation.

Ingredients:

Meatballs:

• 1 pound ground lamb

• 1 yellow onion, finely grated

• 1/3 cup chickpea flour

• 1 teaspoon sea salt

• 1 tablespoon ground turmeric

• 2 teaspoons black pepper, freshly ground

Carrots and Potatoes:

• 1/4 cup avocado oil

• 1 yellow onion, finely chopped

- 1 teaspoon sea salt

- 2 tablespoons ground turmeric

- 2 teaspoons black pepper, freshly ground

- 3 cups water

- 1/2 cup fresh lemon juice

- 4 carrots, peeled and cut into 1-inch rounds

- 4 small gold potatoes, cut into 1-inch cubes

- Chopped parsley, for serving

Directions:

1. To make the meatballs, place all ingredients into a large mixing bowl and mix well using your hands. Form into balls using a tablespoon, place on a plate, and set aside.

2. In a large, deep skillet, add oil to the bottom of the pan and heat to medium heat. Once oil is hot, add in chopped onion and salt. Stir occasionally until golden brown, about 10-15 minutes. Add in ground turmeric and stir to mix well and cook until fragrant, about 1 minute.

3. Add water to the skillet and increase heat to medium-high heat. Add in lemon juice and black pepper. Bring to a boil, then lower heat to maintain a simmer. Add in meatballs and cook for 5 minutes, turning over once for even cooking. Next, add in carrots and potatoes, stirring gently so that they are evenly distributed in the skillet.

4. Bring mixture back up to a boil, then reduce heat to low and keep at a simmer for one hour until the meatballs are done, vegetables are fork-tender, and sauce has reduced down and thickened.

5. Serve hot with chopped parsley on top.

Chocho has been eaten for generations in South American Andean communities, though its high-protein wonders are little known stateside. The legume looks similar to Italian lupini beans when whole. Per cup, choco has 27 grams of protein (most beans such as black and garbanzo beans only have 15). Though it roughly has the same amount of calories as other legumes (238 versus 227-269), it is relatively low-carb (10 grams versus 41-45). When baked, it has a neutral flavor and the consistency of delicate, glutinous rice flour like mochi.

Ingredients:

• 1 tablespoon ground flax seeds

• 1/2 cup gluten-free all-purpose flour

• 1/2 cup chocho flour, available from Five Sun Foods

• 1 tablespoon psyllium husk

• 1/2 teaspoon salt

• 1 tablespoon ground cinnamon

• 1 (4-ounce) container applesauce

- 1 cup coconut sugar

- 3 tablespoons coconut oil

- 1/2 cup almond milk

- 1 1/2 tablespoons vanilla extract

- 1/2 cup raw walnuts, chopped

- 2 cups carrots, shredded by hand

- 1/2 tablespoon baking powder

- 1/2 tablespoon baking soda

- 1 tablespoon white sesame seeds

Directions:

1. Preheat oven to 325°F. Grease a muffin tin.

2. Combine flaxseed, gluten-free flour, chocho flour, psyllium husk, salt, and cinnamon in a medium mixing bowl with a whisk until homogenous.

4. In a separate mixing bowl, combine apple sauce, coconut sugar, coconut oil, almond milk, and vanilla with a whisk until homogenous.

Whether you're making it for breakfast, lunch, or dinner, grab a handful of veggies and your favorite chopsticks and try your hand at this DIY cauliflower sushi.

Ingredients:

• 1 half head of cauliflower

• 1 tablespoon rice wine vinegar

• 1 teaspoon sugar

• 3-4 sheets nori

• assorted veggies and fruit for filling (we used a couple carrots, half of a cucumber, half a mango and an avocado, but use any of your faves you have on hand)

• bamboo sushi rolling mat

• food processor

Instructions:

1. Start by preparing the cauliflower rice. Cut the cauliflower in half (a second time) and remove the thick center stem. Cut or break each half into smaller pieces, trimming off any thicker bits of stem that remain.

2. Place all of the cauliflower pieces into a food processor fit with an S blade and pulse several times until the cauliflower is a small, crumbly texture.

3. Transfer the cauliflower crumble to a microwave-safe bowl, cover with plastic wrap (poke a few holes to allow some steam to escape) and cook on high for three minutes. Remove from microwave and uncover. Mix the sugar with rice vinegar until the sugar starts to dissolve and pour into cauliflower. Stir to combine then set aside to cool while you prepare your fillings.

4. Prepare your veggie and fruit fillings. Remove any unwanted peels or seeds and slice the carrots, cucumber and mango into thin, matchstick-like pieces for easy rolling. Halve and remove the pit and shell of the avocado and cut it into thin slices. Set aside all fillings on a plate to have ready when you assemble the sushi.

5. Lay a sheet of nori on the sushi rolling mat and start to scoop and spread the cauliflower rice onto the nori. You want to cover the nori from edge to edge with a thin even layer of rice, but leave a one-inch space at one end of the nori without rice.

6. Add your fillings, placing them close to the end of the nori where the rice comes all the way to the edge. Lay the pieces in a thin row, and try not to add too much filling as it will make it harder to roll.

7. Now you're ready to start rolling your sushi. Grab a small bowl or glass of water to keep on hand. Place the sushi mat so that the side of the nori with the filling is facing you. Start to roll by pulling up the mat slightly and tucking the row of filling into the first complete roll. Press down with the mat around this to help make a nice tight roll. Continue rolling with the help of the mat and pressing/tucking as you go to keep the roll tight until you get to the end of the nori sheet with the one-inch section without rice. Dab a bit of water on the end of the nori to help it stick to itself and then complete your final roll.

8. Using a clean, sharp knife, cut the sushi into pieces. If your ends are looking a little messy, you can trim these off first to have a nice clean edge. It also helps to wipe off your knife after every one to two slices so that you keep the cuts clean and without bits of cauliflower rice getting onto the nori.

9. Continue this sushi prep and rolling process until you have finished up all of your rice and filling. A half head of cauliflower rice will make about three to four rolls depending on how much you fill them. Then you can dig in!

Get rid of those paprika-sprinkled monstrosities, and replace with our upgraded smoked salmon deviled eggs. Not only are they topped with smoked salmon, but the filling is also packed with smoked salmon (plus some delish extras like lemon zest and Dijon mustard). They're a low-carb treat that's perfect for game day, picnics (LOVE these picnic hacks BTW), and parties, or just to treat yourself to an awesome packed lunch. If you like this recipe — tried our curried pickled eggs too!

Ingredients:

- 6 large eggs

- 3 Tablespoons cream cheese

- 3 Tablespoons mayonnaise

- ½ teaspoon Dijon mustard

- zest of one lemon

- 1 teaspoon lemon juice

- pinch of dried dill

- ¼ teaspoon salt

• 4 ounces good quality smoked salmon, half finely chopped, half sliced into strips (you'll need 12 strips)

• 1 Tablespoon freshly chopped parsley

• 1 Tablespoon freshly chopped chives

• 1/4 teaspoon freshly ground black pepper

Instructions:

1. Place the eggs in a pan of cold water. Bring to the boil and simmer for 10 minutes. Remove from the heat, drain off the hot water, and fill the pan up again with cold water and a cup of ice (this cools the eggs down quickly and aids in removing the egg shell).

2. Tap the eggs, roll to break the shell, and peel off. Slice each egg in half and remove the egg yolks with a teaspoon.

3. Place the egg yolks in a bowl along with the cream cheese, mayonnaise, mustard, lemon juice, lemon zest, salt, dill, and the finely chopped smoked salmon. Blend together with a hand blender until smooth, then transfer the mixture to a piping bag or plastic sandwich bag with the corner cut off (no nozzle needed).

4. Place the cooked egg whites on a serving plate and pipe the salmon mixture into the egg whites. Roll up the salmon strips and push them into the salmon mixture in the eggs. Sprinkle with parsley, chives, and black pepper before serving.

Looking to add a little lean protein to your life without making chicken... again? This cod dish recipe is an easy and elegant meal to prepare that's both healthy and flavorful. A crunchy almond coating adds texture, and the lemon-yogurt dill sauce brings added flavor. Not that there's anything wrong with chicken, but it can show up a lot in the weekly rotation, and that could lead to dinner boredom and burnout. Variety is the spice of life, after all.

Ingredients:

• 5 Tablespoons plain Greek yogurt, divided

• 1 Tablespoon lemon juice

• 3 teaspoons fresh dill, divided, plus extra as garnish (optional)

• salt and pepper to season

• 1/4 cup ground almonds

• 3 Tablespoons grated Parmesan cheese

• 3 Tablespoons breadcrumbs (or almond meal)

• 2 (4-ounce) cod fillets

Instructions:

1. Preheat oven to 400 degrees Fahrenheit. Add a piece of parchment paper to a baking pan and set aside.

2. To make the lemon-yogurt dill sauce, add 3 tablespoons of the Greek yogurt to a small bowl. Add the lemon juice and half the dill. Season with a pinch of salt and stir to combine. Refrigerate until ready to use.

3. Add the almonds to a food processor and pulse until small pieces form. Add the almonds, Parmesan, breadcrumbs, and half the dill to a bowl and toss to combine. Season with a bit of black pepper.

4. Season each piece of the cod with salt and pepper. Place on the parchment-covered baking pan.

5. Use a small brush to apply a thin layer of the remaining yogurt over the fillets. Use your hands to apply the almond mixture over the tops of the fillets, pressing down lightly so the coating sticks.

6. Bake for 9-12 minutes, depending on how thick your fillets are, or until the fish flakes easily.

7. Serve warm with a side of your favorite vegetables, and the lemon-yogurt dill sauce on the side.

Spaghetti s□uash is in season and it's a great low-carb, low-calorie, and gluten-free alternative to pasta.

Ingredients:

– 1 spaghetti s□uash

– extra-virgin olive oil

– salt and pepper, to taste

Instructions:

1. Preheat the oven to 400 degrees F. Cut spaghetti squash in half lengthwise. Use a spoon to remove the seeds. Drizzle with olive oil and season with salt and pepper.

2. Place cut side down in a roasting pan. Bake for 35-40 minutes. Let cool for 5-10 minutes.

3. Using a fork, scrape around the edges of the s□uash to shred your "noodles."

Preheat the oven to 400 degrees F. Cut spaghetti squash in half lengthwise. Use a spoon to remove the seeds. Drizzle with olive oil and season with salt and pepper.

your favorite taco fillings, including steak, are stuffed inside crispy cheddar cheese shells for a beginner recipe that's easy enough to tackle on a weeknight for one person. This recipe might leave you with a little leftover steak... but who's complaining about that? Chop it up and add it to a salad the next day. Be sure to look for a taco seasoning that is low in carbs as some brands sneak in sugar. Customize the toppings to your liking, and let the feasting begin.

Ingredients

• 3/4 cup shredded cheddar cheese, divided

• 1 packet taco seasoning

• 1 New York strip steak

• 1/4 stick butter

• diced tomato, for topping

• sour cream, for topping

• sliced avocado, for topping

• sliced jalapeño, for topping

• lime zest, for topping

Directions

Preheat oven to 375°F. Line a sheet pan with parchment paper or a Silpat. Set out four glasses that are similar in height and rest a wooden cooking spoon over each pair of glasses. These suspended spoons will be used to shape the tortillas.

Divide cheese into three mounds on top of lined sheet pan. Use hand to flatten and spread cheese into circles spaced 1-2 inches apart. Bake for 10-15 minutes, or cheese appears lacy and is golden-brown on the edges.

Use a spatula to carefully drape tortillas over suspended spoons to create tortilla shape. Allow to dry and harden.

Meanwhile, sprinkle taco seasoning over both sides of the steak. You may not use the whole packet.

Preheat a grill or grill pan to medium-high. If using a grill pan, melt butter over the top and allow to brown slightly. For medium rare or medium steak, cook for 2-3 minutes. Rotate steak 90 degrees using a fork, and cook for an additional 2-3 minutes. Flip steak with a fork, and repeat process. Remove steak onto a plate and allow to rest for 10-15 minutes, before slicing into thin strips against the grain.

When it comes to eating salads, we kinda need to be impressed. Salads can be *delicious*, but it takes innovative cooking, tons of flavor, and seasonal ingredients to get our attention. That's one of the reasons we LOVE this winter salad recipe from Most Hungry. Fennel is one of those flavors that feels fresh but is totally in season during the winter months, making it an ideal ingredient for creative recipes around the holidays.

Ingredients:

• Chicken cutlet, breaded and fried

• 1 bulb fennel, finely sliced

• 1 small shallot, finely sliced

• 1-2 blood oranges – supremed, sliced diced... whatever you have the patience for

• 1/4 cup walnuts, toasted and roughly chopped

• Small bunch of thyme

• A few fennel fronds, roughly torn

- Olive oil

- Fresh ground pepper

- Flakey salt

Directions:

So, since you're mainly making a salad here, all you need to do is combine your ingredients in a large bowl, toss everything gently with you hands and make sure to season with some salt and fresh pepper. Then, top with a healthy drizzle of extra virgin olive oil. Taste to make sure your seasoning is all good, then go ahead and add a generous handful of that salad atop one of those perfectly cooked chicken cutlets and eat up!

We never met a meatball we didn't like but if you're following a ketogenic diet, spaghetti and meatballs are usually off the table. Our keto-friendly version topped over zoodles keeps you on plan while savoring one of the old classics.

Ingredients

• 1 lb. ground chicken

• 1/2 cup blanched almond flour

• 1/2 cup grated high quality Parmesan cheese

• 1 tablespoon dried Italian herbs

• 1/2 tablespoon crushed red pepper flakes

• 2 eggs

• 1/2 cup heavy cream

• 1/2 cup grated onion

• 1/2 cup whole milk ricotta cheese

• 1 teaspoon salt

• cracked black pepper

Instructions

1. Preheat oven to 400°F (preferably convection if you have it), and line a sheet pan with parchment paper or aluminum foil.

2. In a medium mixing bowl, stir all of the ingredients except for the chicken together using a fork until well combined.

3. Place ground chicken in a large mixing bowl, and stir in the ricotta mixture with a fork using large circular motions until well incorporated. (Mixture should seem slightly wet.)

4. Using a 1/4 cup measuring cup, scoop balls onto the parchment-lined sheet pan. Try to space them out evenly. It's okay if they touch.

5. Place in oven and roast for 25 minutes, turning pan halfway through.

6. Remove meatballs from oven and serve immediately with the accoutrements of your choice.

We've developed a new fixation on fajitas, and with this recipe we think you will too. Pull out the trusty sheet pan and get ready for a baked rendition of shrimp fajitas. A few simple tricks amp up the flavor in this easy recipe. First, the marinade is quickly blitzed in a blender to emulsify and combine the spices. Then, the veggies go into the oven and start roasting while the shrimp is marinating.

Ingredients:

• 2 limes

• 1 red bell pepper, seeded and julienned

• 1/2 green bell pepper, seeded and julienned

• 1/2 large yellow onion, thinly sliced

• 2 teaspoons plus 1/3 cup canola oil, divided

• 2 garlic cloves

• 1 teaspoon kosher salt

• 1/2 teaspoon dried oregano

• 1/2 teaspoon chili powder

- 1/2 teaspoon sweet paprika

- 1/2 teaspoon cayenne pepper

- 1/4 teaspoon ground cumin

- 1 pound (41/50 size) raw shrimp, de-veined and shelled

- 6 flour tortillas

- Mexican crema, sour cream, or Greek yogurt

Instructions:

1. Preheat the oven to 400°F. Set the sheet pan close by.

2. Juice 1 1/2 of the limes. Cut the other lime half into six wedges and set them aside.

3. Toss the bell peppers and onion into the 2 teaspoons of canola oil until coated. Scatter them onto the sheet pan in a single layer.

4. Pour the lime juice and garlic into a blender, adding in the remaining oil in a steady stream. Add the salt and spices, pulsing once to combine. Marinate the shrimp, tossing to coat in a large zip-seal bag for 15 minutes.

5. Meanwhile, roast the bell pepper and onion for 10 minutes.

6. Remove the shrimp from the marinade. Polka dot the shrimp onto the sheet pan of roasted veggies. Roast for 8 minutes more or until pink and fragrant.

7. Heat some flour tortillas and set out the Mexican crema or sour cream to serve with the lime wedges.

Sure, chicken breasts are healthy and versatile, but let's be real: The thighs are the real winner. They're cheaper, juicier, and more flavorful, yet they're often overlooked. Why not give them the love they deserve? Enter crispy chicken thighs with honey-lemon pan sauce.

Ingredients

• 4 bone-in, skin-on chicken thighs

• salt and pepper, to taste

• 1-2 tablespoons olive oil

• 5-6 cloves garlic, peeled

• 1 tablespoon butter

• juice of half of a lemon

• 1 1/2 tablespoons honey

• 1-2 tablespoons fresh parsley, stems removed and chopped

Directions

Pre-heat the oven to 425 degrees Fahrenheit. Pat chicken thighs dry, and season with salt and pepper on both sides. Drizzle olive oil over the skin sides.

Set a cast-iron skillet or oven-safe pan over medium heat. Cook the chicken thighs, skin-side down, until very browned and crispy, about 15 minutes. Readjust them about 5 minutes through so the fat touches the skillet and coats it with liquid.

This chicken salad has been saved and shared on the social network over 247K times. That inspired us to reach out to the recipe developer to find out what makes it so dang popular and to see what all the fuss is about.

Ingredients

• 2 boneless skinless chicken breasts

• 1/2 teaspoon paprika

• 1/2 teaspoon garlic powder

• 1/2 teaspoon chili powder

• 1/2 teaspoon cumin

• 1 tablespoon olive oil, plus more for pan

• salt and pepper, to taste

• 2 cups romaine lettuce or baby spinach

• 1 large tomato, cut in a large dice

• 1 small red onion, cut in a medium dice

• 1/2 cup cucumber, cut in a half moons

- 2 avocados, sliced

- 1 tablespoon olive oil

- 1 cilantro fresh or dried

- 1/2 teaspoon salt

- 1/2 teaspoon pepper

Directions

Wash and pat the chicken breasts dry.

In a small bowl, mix together the paprika, garlic powder, chili powder, cumin, two large pinches of salt, a few cracks of black pepper, and olive oil.

Evenly sprinkle the spices on each side of the chicken breasts.

Heat a large cast iron pan over medium-high heat. Drizzle in about 1 tablespoon of olive oil. Cook chicken on medium heat, flipping halfway through cook-time, until it's no longer pink in center (approximately 15 minutes, depending on thickness).

Add all the ingredients (except for the chicken and avocado) to a large salad bowl, drizzling the olive oil, and sprinkling the salt, pepper, and cilantro. Toss with tongs.

Remove the chicken and cut diagonally into strips. Place on top of salad along with the sliced avocado, and serve immediately.

While Chinese takeout usually tastes amazing, it's probably out of the question when you've gone Whole30, paleo, or low-carb. However, don't let that dissuade you from trying to cook similar flavors using compliant ingredients at home.

Ingredients

• 1 cup arrowroot

• 1/2 tablespoon ground ginger

• 1 teaspoon granulated garlic

• 1/4 teaspoon ground cinnamon

• 1 teaspoon kosher salt

• 3 pounds boneless, skinless chicken (breast, thighs or combo — we used 2:1 breast/thigh combo), cubed into approximately 1-inch chunks

• 1/2 cup coconut oil

• 3/4 cup coconut aminos

• 1/4 cup coconut sugar

• 1/4 cup toasted sesame oil

• 10-15 dashes Red Boat fish sauce (other brands are fine, but we think Red Boat tastes the best)

• 2 tablespoons minced fresh ginger

• 1 tablespoon minced fresh garlic

• 1 teaspoon crushed red pepper flakes, optional

• 6-10 dried chile de àrbol

• zest and juice of 2 navel oranges

• cauliflower rice or vegetable noodles like zoodles, to serve

• chopped scallion and sesame seeds, to garnish, optional

Directions

In a large mixing bowl, whisk together the arrowroot, ground ginger, granulated garlic, ground cinnamon, and salt. Add the chunks of chicken, coating each piece thoroughly with the arrowroot mixture. Hands (or tongs) are the best tools for this job.

Heat the 1/2 cup of coconut oil on sauté mode of the Instant Pot for a few minutes. Carefully add the chicken to the hot oil, being sure to shake off excess arrowroot mixture beforehand. Stir every few minutes, allowing the chicken to brown upon contact with bottom of Instant Pot.

Once most of the chicken pieces are browned, add the sauce, chiles de àrbol, orange zest and juice; stir to combine.

Cover and switch Instant Pot to high pressure mode for 10 minutes. Make sure vent is closed.

Ingredients

• 1 pound asparagus spears, woody ends removed

• 3 tablespoons olive oil

• 1 tablespoon minced garlic (or 4 cloves garlic, minced)

• 3/4 teaspoon kosher salt

• 1/4 teaspoon fresh cracked black pepper

• 1 1/4 cups shredded mozzarella cheese

Directions

Preheat oven to 425°F. Lightly grease a baking sheet with nonstick cooking oil spray.

Arrange asparagus on baking sheet. Set aside.

In a small bowl mix together olive oil, garlic, salt and pepper.

Drizzle the oil mixture over the asparagus and toss to evenly coat.

Top with mozzarella cheese. Bake for 10-15 minutes until vibrant and just beginning to get tender. Then broil until the cheese becomes golden (about 4-5 minutes).

Adjust salt and pepper, if needed. Serve immediately.

Cooking delicate white fish like Dover sole at home can seem scary (Will it break when you flip it? Did it cook through?). Though it's tempting to just eat out and get your fish fix at a restaurant, if you equip yourself with this simple pan-seared recipe, you'll be flipping fillets confidently in no time.

Ingredients:

• 1 heaping tablespoon olive oil

• salt and pepper, to taste

• 1 fillet of Dover sole

• 1 tablespoon butter

• 1 tablespoon capers, drained

• 1 clove garlic, peeled and smashed

• juice of 1/2 lemon, plus more for serving

• 1/2 teaspoon rosemary sprigs, chopped

• chopped parsley, for serving

Directions:

1. Heat oil in a pan or cast-iron skillet over medium heat.

2. Pat fish dry, then season with salt and pepper on both sides.

3. Add to pan. Sear until cooked through and lightly browned, about 2 minutes on each side, depending on the thickness.

4. Lower heat slightly, and add butter, capers, garlic, and lemon juice (and rosemary, if using), swirling the pan slightly.

5. When butter has melted and begun to brown, turn off heat and spoon the pan sauce over the fish.

6. Top with parsley, and serve immediately with lemon slices/wedge

Settle in for a classic shepherd's pie dinner just like Mom used to make... but better! This filling, comfort dish has been transformed, so it's perfectly Paleo for a healthier, tasty option. Sorry not sorry, Mom. There's nothing complicated here: You'll find beef, veggies, seasonings, and a creamy topping in this crave-worthy comfort food dish that goes Paleo with mashed cauliflower as a topping instead of standard spuds.

Ingredients:

• 4 Tablespoons olive oil, divided

• 1 head cauliflower, stem removed and chopped into small pieces

• 2 cups water

• 1/4 cup white onion, diced

• 1 cup carrot, diced

• 2 garlic cloves, minced

• 1 red bell pepper, seeds and membrane removed, diced

• 2 cups asparagus, cut into 1-inch pieces

- 1 pound ground beef

- 1/2 teaspoon ground cumin

- 1/2 teaspoon coriander

- 1/2 teaspoon salt

- 1/4 teaspoon black pepper

- 1/4 teaspoon red pepper flakes

- paprika, to garnish

Instructions:

1. To make the cauliflower mash: Add 1-1/2 tablespoons olive oil to a large pot over medium heat. When hot, add the cauliflower pieces and cook for 4-5 minutes, or until it begins to turn golden. Add the water, reduce the heat slightly, and cover. Cook for 7-9 minutes or until soft. Drain the cauliflower and reserve the cooking water.

2. Add the cauliflower to a food processor. Add 2 tablespoons of the cooking water and pulse until smooth. Add another 2 tablespoons of the water as needed, and blend to the consistency you like. Set aside.

3. To make the filling: Preheat the oven to 400 degrees Fahrenheit. Add 1-1/2 tablespoons olive oil to a large skillet over medium heat. When hot, add the onion and carrot. Cook until soft. Add garlic, bell pepper, and asparagus to the skillet with the vegetables. Add about 1/4 cup of the remaining cauliflower water to the skillet with the vegetables and cook until they begin to soften.

4. Meanwhile, add 1 tablespoon of olive oil to a second skillet over medium heat. When hot, add the ground beef and cook until browned. When the ground beef is cooked, use a slotted spoon to transfer it to the skillet with the vegetables. Add the cumin, coriander, salt, black, and red pepper to the mixture. Stir to combine.

5. To assemble: Transfer the mixture to a cast iron skillet (or a lightly oiled baking dish if using). Transfer the mashed cauliflower over the top of the mixture and spread it out evenly. Sprinkle the paprika over the top.

6. Bake for about 20 minutes. Serve immediately.

Enter this cauliflower "rice" bowl with flavorful marinated chicken and meaty shiitake mushrooms, then topped with healthy fats from avocado and spicy mayonnaise. Whether you're a lean, mean Keto machine or are simply striving for a low-carb diet, you'll find something to love in this bowl full of tasty textures and temperatures.

Ingredients:

• 1 pound chicken breast, cut into cubes

• 1/4 cup coconut aminos (or soy sauce if you don't mind the sugar. Trader Joe's Soyaki Sauce would also be delicious, but not Keto)

• salt and pepper, to taste

• 1 English cucumber, peeled, deseeded, and sliced into matchsticks

• 1 teaspoon Trader Joe's Yuzu Hot Sauce (or a combination of white vinegar, sesame oil, and a Keto hot sauce)

• 4 Tablespoons mayonnaise

• 3 Tablespoons sriracha, adjusted to desired level of heat

- 3 Tablespoons coconut oil, divided

- 1 pound riced cauliflower

- 8-10 ounces shiitake mushrooms, sliced

- 1 teaspoon ground ginger

- 1 large avocado, sliced

- 1 Tablespoon sesame seeds

Instructions:

1. Prep the chicken: Place chicken in a plastic bag with coconut aminos, salt, and pepper. Mix until chicken is coated, and marinate in the refrigerator for 30 minutes or up to 2 hours.

2. Prep the cucumber slaw: Toss the cucumber matchsticks with yuzu hot sauce. Set aside, keeping cool.

3. Prep the sriracha mayonnaise: Mix mayonnaise and sriracha until completely combined.

4. Heat 1 tablespoon coconut oil in a skillet. Add chicken, and cook until browned and cooked through, about 10 minutes. Use tongs or a spatula to ensure the pieces are cooked on all sides. Set aside.

5. Meanwhile, heat 1 tablespoon coconut oil in a separate skillet. Add cauliflower rice and sauté until softened, about 10 minutes. Halfway through, add salt and pepper. Set aside.

6. In the same skillet as the chicken, heat 1 tablespoon coconut oil, and add mushrooms. Cook until tender, about 10 minutes. Halfway through, add ground ginger, salt, and pepper.

7. Place chicken, mushrooms, cucumber slaw, and sliced avocado over cauliflower rice. Drizzle sriracha mayonnaise and sprinkle sesame seeds on top.

We're huge fans of the low-carb, keto-friendly sous vide egg bites from Starbucks, but as much as we love the bacon-gruyere-filled breakfast, we can't splurge on them everyday of the week. That's why we decided to give it a hacked go at home. These egg bites are totally easy to make-ahead, so you can cook them on a Sunday and reheat them in the microwave throughout the week. You can even mix up the ingredients and try different combinations to keep things interesting.

Ingredients:

• 1/4 cup cottage cheese

• 4 eggs

• 1/4 shredded Monterey jack cheese

• 2 pinches kosher salt

• a few dashes of hot sauce

• nonstick spray, for rimming mason jars

• 4 pieces of bacon, cooked until semi-crispy but still malleable

- 1/4 shredded gruyere cheese, plus more for topping

Need a healthy dish that can cure the darkest of days? Warm, comforting ramen can be easily converted into a low-carb recipe if you replace the traditional wheat noodles with zucchini noodles (or Skinny Pasta noodles) and swap out soy sauce for liquid coconut aminos. Our keto version still has all of your favorite parts of traditional ramen, from the deeply flavored, mushroom-accented broth to the jammy soft-boiled egg and melt-in-your-mouth crispy pork belly. Dress up your bowl with whatever low-carb toppings you like, such as sliced green onion and seaweed sheets, and you'll impress even yourself with a tasty, 'grammable dish that takes less time to make at home than it does to order at a Japanese restaurant.

Ingredients:

• 12 ounces pork belly, cut into 1/4-inch thick slices

• 4 cloves garlic, peeled and grated

• 2 teaspoons grated fresh ginger

• 4 cups chicken bone broth

• 3 tablespoons coconut aminos

• 2 teaspoons chili paste

• 3 1/2 ounces (about 2 heaping cups) shiitake mushrooms, sliced into matchsticks

• salt and pepper, to taste

• 10 ounces zucchini noodles

• 2 to 4 soft-boiled eggs (sliced into halves), to garnish

• 6 sliced green onions (just the crunchy light green part), to garnish

• 6 to 8 nori seaweed sheets, to garnish

Directions:

1. Cook pork belly in a large pan over medium heat until crispy on the outside, about 5 minutes on each side.

2. Turn off the heat and remove pork belly and all but 2 tablespoons of fat from the pot. Allow fat to cool slightly.

3. Return heat to low-medium (fat will still be hot), and cook garlic and ginger, stirring often until fragrant, about 2 minutes.

4. Add bone broth, coconut aminos, chili paste, mushrooms, and salt and pepper to pot. Bring to a boil, then simmer for 10 minutes, stirring occasionally.

5. Add zoodles, and cook until al dente, about 5 minutes.

6. Divide ramen into bowls. Top with eggs, green onion, and seaweed sheets, and serve.

This high-protein alternative to bread is basically a meringue with its yolks added back in to the mixture and baked. Since it is almost 100 percent egg, it does have a slightly eggy flavor, but the fluffiness mimics the texture of traditional bread. From there, add in dried herbs and spices to complement your desired flavor profiles. Think cinnamon for breakfast breads or curry for an Indian open-faced sandwich lunch. The options are endless. Here, we've used ricotta cheese alongside garlic and dried Italian herbs to ensure we accomplish Italy on the palate.

Ingredients:

• 3 eggs, separated

• 3 tablespoons full fat ricotta cheese

• 1/8 teaspoon cream of tartar

• 1/2 teaspoon garlic powder

• 1/2 teaspoon dried Italian herbs

• about 8 tablespoons sugar free pizza or marinara sauce

• 8 ounces part-skim shredded mozzarella cheese

• 24 slices pepperoni

• optional toppings: sliced black olives, diced bell pepper

Directions:

1. Preheat oven to 300°F and prepare a baking sheet by lining it with parchment paper.

2. In a medium mixing bowl, combine the egg whites and cream of tartar.

3. Whip the egg whites with a hand mixer (or by hand or with a stand mixer) until stiff peaks are achieved.

4. In a small mixing bowl, combine the egg yolks with ricotta cheese, garlic powder and dried Italian herbs; stir until thoroughly combined.

5. Gently fold the egg yolk mixture into the egg white mixture by using a spatula to "cut" into the middle and fold over while rotating the bowl after each fold over.

6. Using a 1/4 cup measure, portion 8 (3-inch) rounds of fluffy egg white mixture onto prepared baking sheet. Each round should be about 1/2-inch thick.

7. Bake cloud breads for 30-35 minutes, until golden brown. Allow to cool and rest for at least 30 minutes before building pizzas.

8. Adjust oven temp to 350°F.

9. Build pizzas by spreading about 1 tablespoon of pizza sauce, plenty of cheese, and 3 slices of pepperoni (and/or any other toppings).

10. Place in oven for 15 minutes or until cheese is melted and slightly browned.

11. Serve immediately.

Two of my favorite food groups—eggs and toast—unite in this take on the playful dish also known as toad in the hole or, more simply, egg in toast. Fancy it up by adding a handful of spinach along with the cheese or topping with salsa or pesto. Watch carefully as you cook the crust, and don't raise the heat higher than medium: The goal is for the crust to brown and the egg to set simultaneously. If you are using a frozen crust, stamp out the holes while it is slightly frozen to keep the crusts from tearing. Save the crust rounds for making crostini or breadcrumbs.

Ingredients:

• 1 Cali'flour Pizza Crust

• 2 teaspoons ghee or unsalted butter

• 2 large eggs

• sea salt and freshly ground black pepper

• 1/4 cup (30 grams) shredded cheddar or other melting cheese

• 2 strips bacon, cooked and crumbled (optional)

• sriracha or other hot sauce (optional)

Directions:

1. Using a pizza wheel, cut the crust in half. Using a 3-inch cookie cutter or the top of a thin drinking glass, stamp out a hole from the middle of each crust half.

2. Melt the ghee in a 12-inch skillet that has a lid over medium heat (or cook the baskets one at a time in a smaller skillet).

3. Using a metal spatula, carefully place the crusts in the skillet, then crack an egg directly into each hole and season with salt and pepper. Scatter the cheese on the exposed crust, cover the pan, and cook until the whites are set and the cheese is melted, about 3 minutes.

4. Using the metal spatula, remove from the pan to plates and top with the bacon and hot sauce, if using.

As far as I'm concerned, almost anything with toasted sesame oil is going to be good, and that's certainly true of this ginger-scented halibut and- mushroom parcel. Like the previous papillote recipe, this serves two but could be easily scaled up for a bigger crowd (It seems like all my friends want to come over when I'm making it).

Ingredients:

• 2 medium shiitake, oyster, or maitake mushrooms, thinly sliced

• 2 (6-ounce) halibut fillets, skin removed

• flaky sea salt and cracked black pepper

• 1/2 teaspoon grated lemon zest

• 1/2 teaspoon grated fresh ginger

• 2 scallions, thinly sliced

• 1 teaspoon coconut aminos

• 1/2 teaspoon toasted sesame oil, plus more for drizzling

• 4 lemon slices

Directions:

1. Preheat the oven to 400°F. Lay out two 9×11-inch sheets of parchment paper on a flat surface.

2. Place the sliced mushrooms in the lower third of each parchment sheet. Season the halibut fillets generously with salt and pepper and place them on top of the mushrooms.

3. Divide the lemon zest, ginger, scallions, coconut aminos, sesame oil, and lemon slices evenly between the fillets.

Did you grow up eating Brussels sprouts gratin — a bubbly, cheesy baked casserole loaded with a breadcrumb topping? It's not exactly low-carb, which is a problem if you're on a diet like keto. To curb our craving, we made the indulgent recipe over and developed this rich and satisfying three-cheese Brussels sprouts side dish. It happens to comply with the ketogenic diet or any other low-carb eating plan. It's a one-pot dish that can be prepared over the stovetop (rather than the oven), which helps clear space during Thanksgiving or other holidays when you need to prioritize that giant turkey or ham.

Note: This dish can easily be made a couple of days ahead, covered and stored in the refrigerator. Be sure to use an oven-proof skillet or Dutch oven to keep it in one pot if you wish (a casserole dish would also work just fine but negates our one-pot claim). Cover, and re-heat in a 375°F oven for an hour and then uncovered for another 15 minutes.

Ingredients

• 3-4 tablespoons extra virgin olive oil

• 2 pounds Brussels sprouts, halved or quartered depending on size

• 1/2 teaspoon kosher salt

• 4-6 ounces bacon, cut into lardon size (1/4-inch pieces)

• 1 cup diced onion

• 1 1/2 to 2 cups heavy cream

• 1/2 cup sour cream

• 8 ounces grated smoked gouda cheese

• 8 ounces grated low-moisture, part-skim mozzarella cheese

• 4 ounces crumbled feta cheese, for garnish

• 1 teaspoon garlic salt

• freshly ground black pepper

Directions

Heat 3-4 tablespoons olive oil in a large, shallow skillet or Dutch oven over high heat.

Once oil is hot, carefully place the Brussels sprouts into the pan without stirring initially. Cook the sprouts for about 15 minutes, stirring very infrequently so the sprouts char on at least a couple sides. Remove sprouts; set aside.

Add the bacon to the pan; sauté for about 5 minutes, stirring constantly, until bacon is slightly crispy.

Remove bacon onto a paper towel-lined plate; set aside.

Reduce heat to medium. Add the onion to the bacon fat in the skillet. Sauté for 5 more minutes, stirring often, or until onions have softened and caramelized a little.

Add the heavy cream, sour cream, gouda, mozzarella, and feta; stir to combine. Reduce heat to medium-low once cheese melts.

Transfer the Brussels sprouts back to the skillet with the cheese sauce; stir to combine. If the sauce seems too thick, stir in more heavy cream little by little. Season with the garlic salt and freshly ground black pepper to taste.

Garnish the Brussels sprouts with the reserved bacon. Serve immediately.

Low Carb Mini Quiche Cups

If you weren't convinced by the 12 delightful cauliflower recipes from yesterday, then these Cauliflower Quiche Cups will definitely pi?ue your interest. This veggie packed, low carb tart is perfect any time of the day. Not only is it easy to grab and go, it's packed with all the vitamins and nutrients needed to help you beat that afternoon food coma!

Ingredients:

• 1/2 of a cauliflower (medium sized)

• 2 packed cups of washed and cut kale

• 1/2 cup shredded mozzarella cheese, plus more for garnishing

• 1/4 cup sun dried tomatos

• 1/4 cup egg whites

• 1/8 cup cottage cheese

• sunflower seeds for garnish

Tools

• Food processor

• Mini tart pan

Direction

As usual, get the oven started and preheat to 375 degrees F. Then, we'll prepare the cauliflower.

Cut off the stem of the cauliflower. Then cut the cauliflower into small florets. Put it in the food processor and pulse until it looks like grains of rice. Remove from the food processor and microwave for 6 minutes. You don't need to cover it.

While the cauliflower is microwaving, you can prepare more of the filling. In a food processor, pulse the kale until it becomes large chunks. Then, add in the sun dried tomatoes and pulse. When it's all shredded, add in the cheese and repeat until everything is shredded.

When the cauliflower is done microwaving, add in the kale mixture to the cauliflower. Pour in the egg whites, cottage cheese, and mix together with a spoon.

After your mixture is complete, spray your tart pan with cooking spray and then begin filling it! When you're done filling all the cups, garnish with cheese and sunflower seeds.

When they're all done, pop into the oven for about 20 minutes, or until the tops begin to brown.

We love that golden brown crust. Yum!

Mexican-style hot dogs in lettuce wraps are fun to serve, flavorful, and yes, a little lower in carbs, because the standard buns get ditched. When you're planning your next cookout or balcony barbecue, wrap those dogs in lettuce leaves and toss together some Mexican-inspired toppings for a twist on tradition.

Don't forget the sour cream, salsa, lime juice to squeeze over the top, a sprinkle of hot sauce, and Cotija cheese to crumble too. Use Bibb lettuce as the bun since the leaves aren't so big that they take over your dog yet still wrap around the hot dog and toppings. Buy an extra package of dogs for your next cookout, because second helpings are practically guaranteed.

Ingredients:

• 6 hot dogs, cooked

• 6 Bibb lettuce leaves, washed and dried

• 1 (15-ounce) can black beans, drained

• 1 (15-ounce) can corn kernels, drained and rinsed

• 6 ounces (about 1 heaping cup) shredded cheddar cheese

• 2 jalapeño peppers, sliced into rounds, seeds removed

• 1-2 avocados, sliced

• sour cream, to dollop (optional)

• salsa, to spoon over the hotdogs (optional)

E�uipment:

• cooking string or thin ribbon

Instructions:

1. Place one cooked hot dog in the center of a lettuce leaf.

2. Spoon the remaining ingredients over the top and enjoy.

Steamed Sea Bass with Broccoli, Mushrooms, and Summer Squash

RECIPE

he steam gives the fish a moist and tender texture and cooks the vegetables perfectly — not too crispy, not too soggy. And because you cook all the ingredients in aluminum foil, cleanup is easy and super fast. Twenty minutes after you pop this concoction in the oven, unwrap the foil and announce, "Dinner's ready."

Ingredients

• 6 (4-ounce) sea bass filets

• 3/4 teaspoon salt

• 1/4 teaspoon ground white or black pepper

• 1 tablespoon chopped fresh basil or parsley

• 1/2 cup thinly sliced broccoli florets

• 1/2 cup sliced fresh mushrooms

• 1/2 thinly sliced yellow squash

• 1 tablespoon reduced-calorie margarine*

- 6 lemon wedges

Instructions

1. Preheat the oven to 450°F. Tear off a sheet of heavy-duty aluminum foil, one large enough to hold all ingredients comfortably (about 2 feet long). Coat the foil with fat-free cooking spray.

2. Put the fish in the center of the foil and sprinkle with half of the salt, pepper, and basil or parsley. Top with the broccoli, mushrooms, and squash. Sprinkle with the remaining salt, pepper, and basil or parsley. Dot with pieces of the margarine.

3. Bring together the long sides of the foil and fold down tightly over the fish. Fold up the short sides of the foil.

4. Put the packet on a baking sheet and bake until the fish is just opaque, 18 to 20 minutes. (It's okay to open the packet to check that the fish is opaque all the way through.)

This soup is a staple in our house. Not only is it easy to make, but it's also filled with flavor and is oh-so-satisfying. Why? Because avocado . . . and lots of it! I just love this soup, rain or shine, and I know you will too.

Ingredients:

• 2 quarts Whole30-compliant chicken broth or chicken bone broth

• 1 can (14.5 ounces) Whole30-compliant diced tomatoes

• 1 medium white onion, finely diced

• 1 jalapeño, seeded and finely diced

• 3 cloves garlic, minced

• 1 tablespoon chipotle powder or regular chili powder

• 1 teaspoon ground cumin

• 1 teaspoon dried oregano

• 1/2 teaspoon salt

• 1/2 teaspoon black pepper

• 4 (2 pounds) boneless, skinless chicken breasts

- 1/2 cup chopped fresh cilantro

- 1/2 cup fresh lime juice, plus lime wedges for serving

- 3 avocados, halved, pitted, peeled, and diced

Directions:

1. In a 6-quart slow cooker, stir together the broth, tomatoes, onion, jalapeño, garlic, chipotle powder, cumin, oregano, salt, and pepper. Add the chicken.

2. Cover and cook on low for 8 to 10 hours or on high for 4 to 5 hours.

3. Use tongs to transfer the chicken to a cutting board. Use two forks to shred the chicken. Return the chicken to the cooker and stir in the cilantro and lime juice.

4. Top servings with avocado and serve with lime wedges.

This recipe certainly looks attractive, and thankfully, it's nutritious too. "I am a big advocate of protein in every meal, so eggs in muffin form are a no-brainer, especially since you can customize them with any variety of veggies, meats, or cheeses, and they freeze and reheat like a breeze," she explains. Her colorful egg muffins just so happen to fit in your busy lifestyle too, which she thinks attributes to the recipe's success. "I'm all about quick, easy, make-ahead meals (hello, two kids ages two and under!) and a hearty breakfast is critical to kick-off the morning and keep my energy up," she adds.

Ingredients:

• nonstick cooking spray

• 12 large eggs

• 1/4 cup milk

• 1 cup fresh spinach, chopped

• 3/4 cup cherry tomatoes, ⬚uartered

• 1/2 cup onion, finely diced

• 1/2 teaspoon kosher salt

- 1/2 teaspoon freshly cracked black pepper

- sliced avocado, for serving

- salsa, for serving

- crumbled cotija or feta cheese, for serving

Directions:

1. Preheat the oven to 350°F. Grease a muffin pan with cooking spray. We used a Silpat Muffin Mold, because it's nonstick.

2. In a large bowl, whisk together the eggs and milk.

3. Stir in the spinach, tomatoes and onions, salt, and pepper.

4. Divide the mixture evenly between the 12 muffin pan cups (a spring-form ice cream scooper helps).

5. Bake the muffins for 20 to 25 minutes, or until the egg is fully cooked.

6. Remove the muffins from the oven and let them cool for 5 minutes in the pan. They may be puffy and lopsided, but they will deflate evenly as they cool. Use a knife to loosen the muffins from the cups, if necessary.

7. Top each muffin with sliced avocado, a dollop of salsa, and a sprinkling of cheese, then serve.

We replaced the traditional breadcrumbs in the meatballs with blanched almond meal as a binder. Almost any nut flour would work really well in its place. Other than that, we amped up the keto-ness by stuffing the balls with cheese and flavored a sugar-free jarred marinara with diced pancetta, which is always a good idea. You literally throw everything into the Instant Pot and approximately 15 minutes later, dinner is on the table for the entire family.

Ingredients:

• 1 egg

• 1/2 cup whole milk

• 1/2 cup blanched almond meal

• 1/2 cup grated parmesan cheese

• 1/2 teaspoon crushed red pepper

• freshly ground black pepper

• 1 pound mild, uncured Italian sausage (removed from casings if purchased in links; we bought loose sausage from the butcher)

• 1 pound lean ground beef

• 1/2 cup shredded part-skim low-moisture mozzarella, plus more (to garnish)

• 2 ounces diced pancetta

• 2 cloves garlic, roughly chopped

• 1/2 (25-ounce) jar no-added-sugar marinara sauce

• 1/4 cup chicken stock

• zoodles, heated (for serving)

• basil, chiffonade (to garnish)

Directions:

1. In a large mixing bowl, whisk together the egg, milk, almond meal, grated parmesan, crushed red pepper flakes, and freshly ground black pepper (as much or as little as you would like). Let it sit for about 5 minutes to allow almond meal to absorb liquid.

2. Add the sausage and ground beef. Using your hands, mix the ground meat mixture into the wet ingredients until thoroughly combined.

3. Have a baking sheet ready for your meatballs. Fill a 1-cup measuring cup lightly (between 3/4 cup and 1 cup is good). Turn meat out into your hands and flatten it out into a patty.

4. Add about 1 tablespoon shredded mozzarella in the middle of the patty and close patty around the cheese, into a ball shape. Set aside on baking sheet and repeat until all the meat is completed.

5. Select the sauté function on the Instant Pot. Add the diced pancetta and garlic cloves; sauté for about 5 minutes, stirring occasionally.

6. Add the jar of marinara sauce to the Instant Pot. Then use the chicken stock to clean out the tomato sauce jar by sealing and shaking; add stock to Instant Pot and stir to combine.

7. Place raw meatballs into the sauce. Cover, close, and be sure to switch vent to sealing mode. Cook on high pressure for 7 minutes.

8. Once cycle completes, let the pressure release naturally for 10 minutes.

Ingredients

- 4 eggs, separated

- 1/2 teaspoon cream of tartar

- 2 ounces cream cheese, slightly softened

- 2 1/2 tablespoons monk fruit sweetener, divided

- 2 1/2 tablespoons ground cinnamon, divided

Directions

Preheat the oven to 300°F. Line two baking pans with parchment paper.

Add the egg whites and cream of tartar to a stand mixer and mix on high until stiff peaks form. Set aside.

In another bowl, add the cream cheese, 1/2 tablespoon monk fruit sweetener, and 1/2 tablespoon cinnamon. Blend and add one egg yolk at a time until incorporated.

Gently fold the egg yolk mixture into the egg white mixture, careful not to deflate the whites.

Use about 1/4 cup of the mixture per piece of bread. Spoon into 4- to 5-inch rounds on the lined pans, about 1 inch thick.

Bake for 10-12 minutes or until lightly golden.

As the bread bakes, combine the remaining monk fruit sweetener and cinnamon in a bowl.

When the bread is done, remove from the oven and brush the tops lightly with water. Sprinkle the sweetener-cinnamon mixture over each. Serve once cooled.

It doesn't take more than a little olive oil and a pinch of salt to make Brussels sprouts shine, but if you're looking for an easy upgrade we've got one you need to try. We'd like to introduce you to our smashed sprouts recipe — a cheesy, crispy, slightly spicy spin on the usual roasted version that will also fit right into your keto and gluten-free diets. It doesn't involve a lot of ingredients or time, and you can prep most of it in advance. It's our favorite new method for packing in those cruciferous veggies. Top it with a fried egg or alongside your favorite protein, or simply serve on a bed of brown rice to keep things vegetarian.

Ingredients:

• 2 pounds Brussels sprouts, cleaned and trimmed

• 1/4 cup olive oil

• 1 tablespoon apple cider vinegar

• 1 teaspoon kosher salt, plus more for

• 1 teaspoon red chili pepper flakes

• 8 ounces shredded mozzarella cheese

- 1/4 cup grated parmesan cheese

- 1/2 a lemon, quartered

Directions:

1. Blanch the Brussels sprouts. Fill a large bowl with ice and water and set nearby, along with a slotted spoon.

2. Fill a large stock pot with water and add enough kosher salt that the water tastes like sea water.

3. Bring it to a boil and add your Brussels sprouts. Allow to cook until just fork-tender, approximately 10 minutes.

4. Using the slotted spoon, carefully transfer the sprouts to the ice water until they're just cool enough to handle — don't allow them to sit in the water.

5. Drain into a colander and pat dry with a clean dish towel.

6. Season and smash them. Preheat your oven to 450°F and line two rimmed sheet pans with parchment paper.

7. In a large bowl, mix together the olive oil, vinegar, salt, and chili pepper flakes. Add the Brussels sprouts and toss gently to combine.

8. Spread them out across the two sheet pans and use a drinking glass or a jar to "smash" each one so that it fans out. You don't want to completely flatten them; we're just looking for some more surface area to hold the cheese.

9. Roast them up. Sprinkle the mozzarella over each sprout, followed by a pinch of the parmesan.

10. Place in the oven until the cheese is brown and bubbly, approximately 10 minutes.

11. Pile them into a serving dish with a squeeze of the lemon or portion onto plates and enjoy.

Fettucine Alfredo is one of the most beloved comfort food dishes in America, but it's not exactly compatible with most diets (unless it's made with zoodles!). That's what inspired us to make a version that is compliant with vegan, gluten-free, low-carb, and keto diets

Ingredients

• 1 cup roasted macadamia nuts

• 1 cup hot water, plus more as needed

• 1/2 cup nutritional yeast

• zest and juice of 1/2 lemon, or more to taste

• 1/2 teaspoon garlic salt

• 4 tablespoons extra virgin olive oil, divided

• 4 zucchini, ends cut off

• parsley, chopped, to garnish

• 1/4 cup roasted macadamia nuts, chopped, to garnish (optional)

• freshly ground black pepper, to garnish.

Instructions

1. In a high-speed blender, add macadamia nuts and hot water. Allow to sit for 5 minutes. Once softened add nutritional yeast, lemon zest and juice, garlic salt, 2 tablespoons of olive oil. Blend until completely smooth. Taste and adjust seasoning if needed.

2. Spiralize zucchini onto a cutting board or bowl. If you don't have a spiralizer, try using a cheese grater or potato peeler instead.

3. In a sauté pan, heat 2 tablespoons of oil over medium-high heat. Add spiralized zucchini.

4. Cook until wilted and bright green (a few minutes), seasoning with garlic salt.

5. Pour in sauce. Toss to coat, and allow it to heat through for a few minutes.

6. Transfer zoodles to plates.

7. Garnish with parsley, chopped macadamia nuts, and black pepper.

You may think something like cauliflower rice or a cauliflower keto bowl is Pinterest's top cauli recipe. Well, think again. While those dishes are oh-so-trendy, the top spot actually belongs to a way more accessible and comforting food. Saved 281K times and counting, Bang Bang Cauliflower from Kirbie's Cravings features panko-coated florets that are baked until crispy and then coated in a spicy-sweet sauce. Talk about the easiest way to coax yourself into eating more cruciferous veg.

Ingredients:

• 1/2 head of cauliflower cut into bite-sized florets

• 2 large eggs whisked with 1 teaspoon kosher salt

• 2 cups panko bread crumbs, Kikkoman brand preferred for even baking

• 2 tablespoons sweet chili sauce, preferably without chili seeds

• 2 teaspoons hot sauce, like sriracha

• 1/4 cup mayonnaise

• 1 tablespoon honey

• 1 tablespoon fresh parsley, finely chopped, to garnish (optional)

• cayenne, to garnish (optional)

Directions:

1. Preheat oven to 400°F.

2. Dip cauliflower pieces in egg and then roll in panko until fully coated and then place on a baking sheet lined with parchment paper (we lined it with a cooling rack to maximize crispiness around all sides). You may need to use your fingers to press on the coating to help it to stick to the cauliflower bites. Repeat until all cauliflower is coated.

3. Bake for about 20 minutes or until coating is dark golden brown and crunchy.

4. While cauliflower is cooking, make the bang bang sauce. Add all ingredients into a small bowl and whisk until uniform and no mayonnaise lumps remain.

5. Drizzle over finished cauliflower, reserving additional sauce for dipping. Garnish with fresh parsley and/or cayenne if desired.

CONCLUSION

For the person who needs structure in their diet, limiting starchy, sugary carbs will help cut calories and allow for weight loss. And focusing on proteins and fats that are plant-based is the healthy and smart thing to do.

For your long-term health, you have to move on from the initial Atkins 20 diet. It's the later phases of the diet, especially the Atkins 40, that give you the variety of foods that are important for health. You have to exercise and keep portions small while you start eating nuts, seeds, beans, fruits, starchy vegetables, and whole grains again.